NO PAIN IN YOUR MUSCLES

DISCOVER THE SCIENCE BEHIND THE PAIN OF THE MUSCLE AND WHAT YOU CAN DO TO GET RELIEF!

ANDREW SLEEVEON

NO PAIN IN YOUR MUSCLES
Copyright © 2016 by Andrew Sleeveon

TABLE OF CONTENTS

Chapter One: Introduction 4

Causes Of Muscular Pain 5

What Is DOMS? 7

Chapter Two: How To Relieve Muscle Pain After Exercise 9

Other Methods To Relieve Muscle Pain 11

Advantages Of Topical Medication 12

Downside Of Topical Medication 13

Checking On Your Health - Living With Muscle Pain 13

Chapter Three: Useful Of Compression Sleeves 15

What Are Knee Sleeves? 17

Can Knee Sleeves Help Reduce Pain From Your Injuries? 19

How Can A Knee Sleeve Help Your Injury? 20

Chapter Four: What is SleeveON 21

How Does Compression Sleeves Help You? 22

Who Is This Suitable For? 23

CHAPTER ONE:
INTRODUCTION

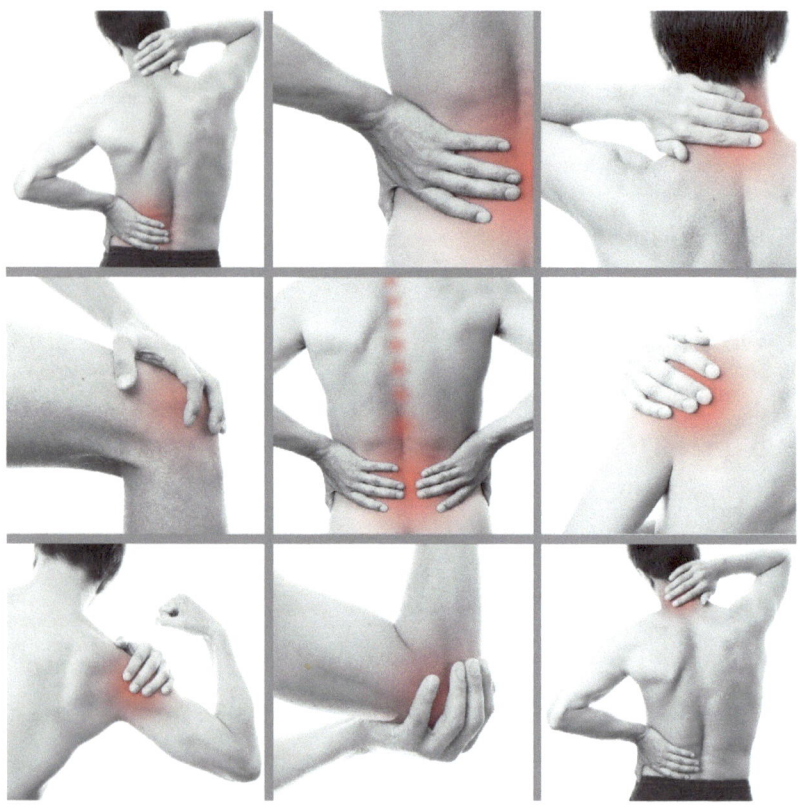

Throughout history, weight lifters have long been vexed by the muscle pain that often accompanies intense workouts. I once saw a very funny comedian who remarked that weight lifting was funny because the only way to know that you've worked out properly is to be so sore that you are unable to move the following day. Then you know what Delayed

Onset Muscle Soreness is like. Discover the science behind the pain and what you can do to get relief!

CAUSES OF MUSCULAR PAIN

- Improper posture.
- Musculoskeletal misalignment - The muscles and bones may be misaligned due to twisting, injury etc.
- Trauma - Repetitive injury.
- Mental and physical stress.
- Muscular overuse due to improper exercise or rigorous labor.

In this book, I will explain what **DOMS** is, why it happens, and what the research shows on how to help ease the pain.

The scientific name for muscle pain after exercise is Delayed Onset Muscle Soreness (DOMS) which typically occurs 12-48 hours after a new workout routine is adopted, after a substantial increase in the duration of exercise, or after abrupt change in athletic activities.

For me, no matter how long I have been exercising, my legs always kill me two days after squats. Part of the reason is, as much as I love to workout, I hate squat days. There are those blessed few who just love crawling out of the squat rack and throwing up in the trash can before the next set (and that's if you do it right).

As much as I hate to admit this, if I could find a reason to "miss" such a workout, I would. It isn't that I have huge legs and don't think that I need to. It isn't just fun for me. I get no "joy in mudville" when I know it is leg day.

I tend to always find a way to make it into a leg press day instead. I can push a lot more weight that way and feel better. I just haven't gotten anymore size in my legs by doing them. I know I have to just suck it up and squat before I will get any larger.

WHAT IS DOMS?

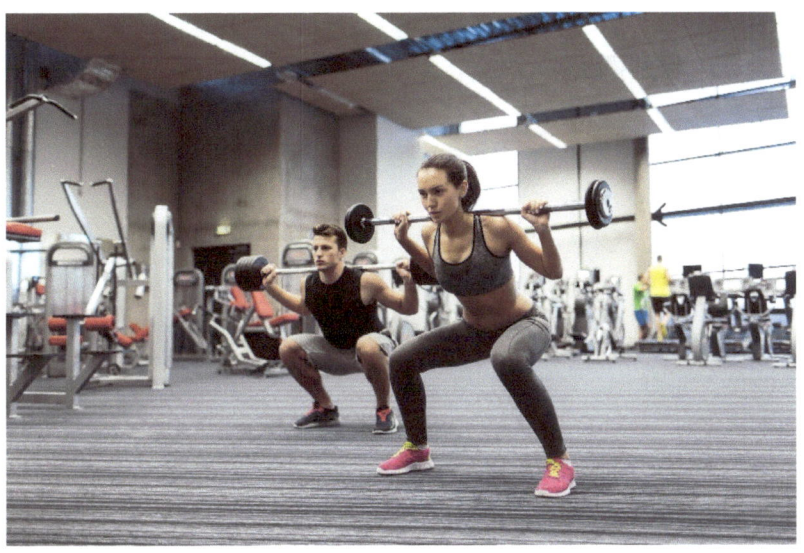

Delayed onset muscle soreness (DOMS) is very familiar to most of us who have been working out for any length of time. Usually, it really only happens when we take an extended break from our workout routine. It also happens when we start using a new piece of exercise equipment.

Any "new" thing that challenges our bodies is a good thing but we can, and usually pay for it. We have all experienced our days of soreness but what causes it and what can I do to speed up my recovery?

DOMS describes a phenomenon of muscle pain and

soreness that is felt 12-48 hours following exercise, particularly at the beginning of a new exercise program, after a change in sports activities, or after a dramatic increase in the duration or intensity of exercise and subsides over the next few days.

If you experience pains in your muscles even when there is no change in your exercises or workout routine, you may actually have a more serious muscle or joint condition or even a serious injury. Muscle pain should always nearly disappear within a few weeks of adopting a new workout program or exercise.

Muscle pain occurs because of little tears that form in the muscle during intense exercise. These little tears gradually heal causing the size and strength of your muscles to increase. The tearing and healing process is part of an adaption process that leads to greater strength and endurance.

CHAPTER TWO:
HOW TO RELIEVE MUSCLE PAIN
AFTER EXERCISE

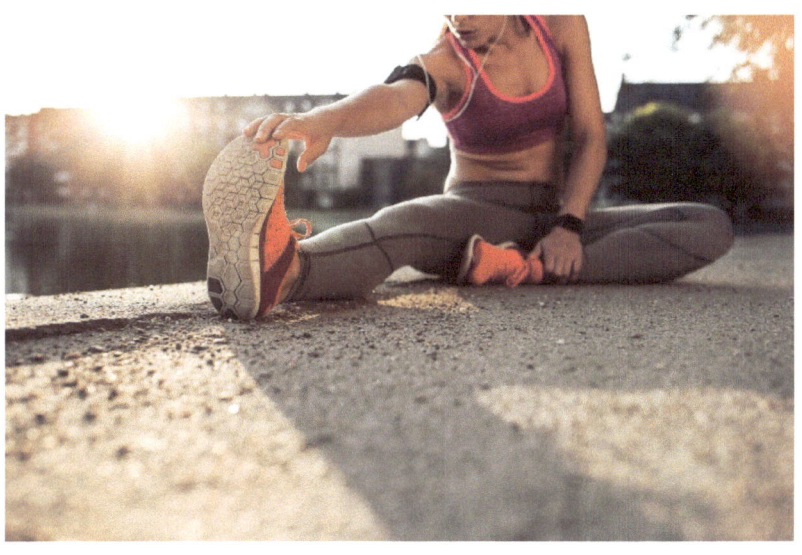

Muscular pain can start with a simple strain or sprain, and increasing to excruciating aches. It is often accompanied by headache, sleeplessness, swelling and even fever, which are just the side-effects.

Amino Acids - These are very inexpensive and can be purchased at your local vitamin store for less than $7 for a 15-day supply. You can choose between liquid and powder tablets but the liquid tablets tend to dissolve faster than the powdered, and are also usually less expensive

Fish Oil - Fish oil contains Omega 3 fatty acids and will reduce inflammation in the joints as well as shorten the length of your muscle pain. This can be purchased very inexpensively at your local vitamin store or even your local grocery store. In addition to relieving pain in your muscles, fish oil will also reduce acne and improve the appearance of your skin.

Aspirin - This is a tried and true pain reliever. 2-4 aspirin tablets taken a few hours after a workout will help reduce DOMS.

Stretching - Performing a few minutes of stretching before a workout or sports activity will not only help eliminate later muscle pain, but will also help prevent serious injuries. 5 minutes of good, solid stretching per hour of exercise is recommended for your normal workout routines and 10 minutes for new exercises or routines or before heavy lifting sets.

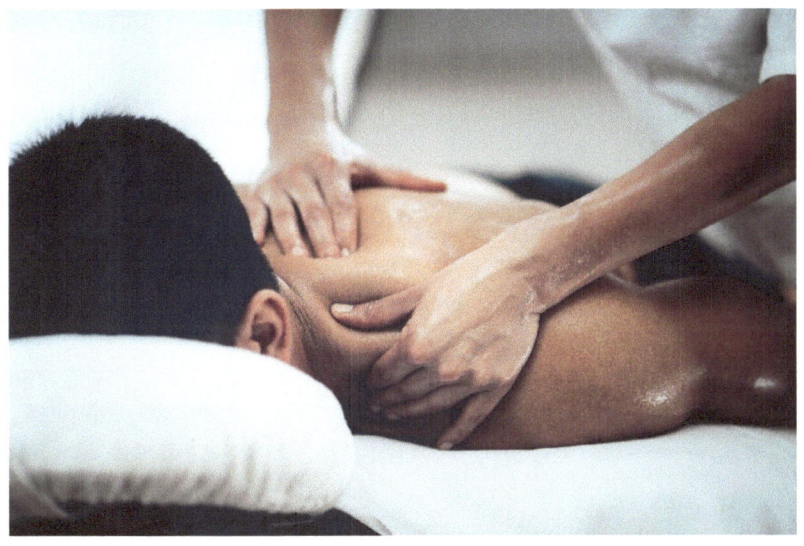

Various Therapies - Many types of therapies are practiced to cure pain in the muscle. They include: exercise, yoga, physiotherapy, heat therapy, oral pills, and ointments. Of these, exercise and yoga have to be taken more cautiously as they involve more twisting and turning which may increase the muscle stress instead of alleviating it. Physiotherapy demands multiple sessions and skilful expertise and is time and money-consuming. Heat therapy works only for certain sprains, and must also be undertaken carefully.

Topical Medication - So, what is the best pain reliever for muscle pain? The best approach is the topical medication or the application of creams, ointments, oils, balm or gels to relieve muscle pain. A few drops of herbal ointment or oil applied tenderly with your fingertips on the affected area might go a long way in removing the pain. Balm or ointment application is the sure-cure for muscle pain relief as it is not only economical, but also readily available and brings immediate relief.

ADVANTAGES OF TOPICAL MEDICATION

Topical ointment application is highly effective as: Ointments are easily absorbed and penetrate deep into the muscle fibers, acting upon them.

Ointments get to the source of the pain very quickly and relax the muscles.

Muscle pain often leads to inflammation or swelling which is due to the accumulation of fluids and toxins. Ointments lubricate the cell walls to eject the toxins and make them absorb the vital medication.

Creams or ointments remove the stiffness from the affected area by lubrication, quickening the relief process.

The only downside to these topical medication that works fast to stop muscle pain, is its side effects which is harmful to our health. The good news is, studies have shown that a number of natural herbs work as effectively as this topical medication, but comes with zero side effects.

Natural Topical Creams - Natural herbs are the best remedy for muscle pain as they are easily available and extracted from our earth's forest reserves. Studies have proven homeopathic muscle pain relievers to include Menthol, Naja, Phosphorus, MSM, Ignatia and many more of such powerful ingredients which do not only have the ability to act fast on providing pain relief, but are also 100% safe to your skin and body.

CHECKING ON YOUR HEALTH - LIVING WITH MUSCLE PAIN

Your muscles represent a significant portion of your body, and that means that there are lots of different physical issues that can cause muscle pain. If you haven't been to the doctor for a while, and your pain is significant enough that you can't seem to move, it's never a bad plan to visit. Remember, aging itself can cause muscle pain as well, so there may be a perfectly understandable cause that is simply something you hadn't considered before.

For you to overcome your own muscle pain, you need to react to that pain the same way that you would react to muscle pain caused by exercise, exertion, or even sleeping wrong:

- Stretch often and make sure you're moving around.
- Hydrate and eat healthy to nourish the muscles.
- Exercise when you can so as to keep your muscles loose.
- Get plenty of rest and make sure you're sitting and standing with good posture.

You should also consider massages and other calming ways to workout the muscles. Anxiety may cause muscle pain, but the pains still relate directly to the exact same issues that cause muscle pain and discomfort in those without anxiety.

CHAPTER THREE:
USEFUL OF COMPRESSION SLEEVES

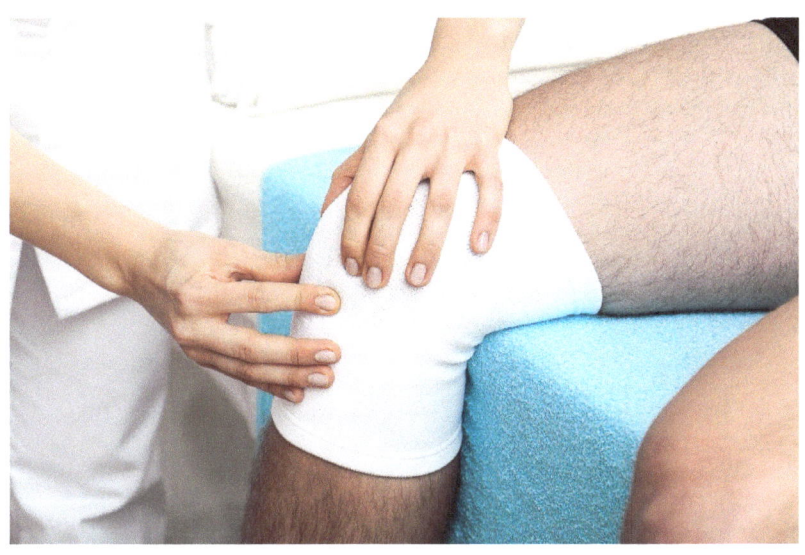

You have probably seen people at races or running around the streets that have those compression sleeves on. Maybe you have thought to yourself, "Does this really work?" or "I wonder if this would help my shin splints or calf cramps?"

To really understand how compression sleeves work, it's important to have a basic understanding of how blood flows through the body. The heart pumps oxygen containing blood to our extremities and working muscles through arteries. Once the cells use the oxygen and other nutrients from the blood, the then deoxygenated blood, along with lactic acid and other waste products enter the veins to be taken back to the heart. Once the blood gets back to the heart, it's oxygenated from the lungs and the process is repeated.

Keeping oxygenated blood flowing to the muscles is important for performance. The more oxygen the cells have, the better they will function. During exercise, the body produces lactic acid as a waste product. If this lactic acid is not removed from the muscles, it can contribute to soreness and decreased ability to perform. Another factor in decreased performance is muscle fatigue. Muscular vibration during physical activity contributes to fatigue. Think about how much shock and vibration is going through your leg muscles as you pound pavement with 3-5 times your body weight while running. Over time, those little vibrations of the muscles add up and they become fatigued.

Compression sleeves provide graduated compression, meaning the compression is higher (tighter) at the foot and ankle, and lower (looser) as it moves up the calf and lower leg. This type of compression helps to fight the effects of gravity and assist the body in venous return (deoxygenated blood flowing back to the heart).

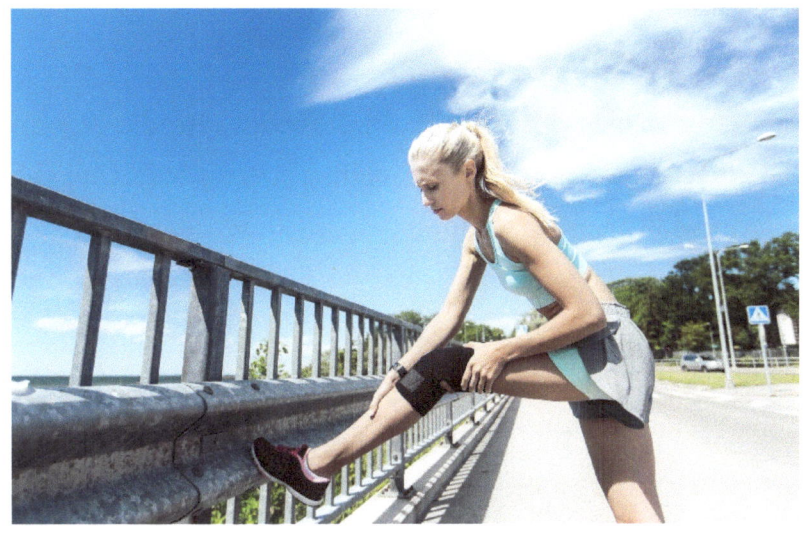

Knee sleeves are designed to protect the knee from future injury or risk of damage. This protection is especially important for knees put under great daily pressure (running, jumping, weightlifting).

Knee sleeves also add a valuable compression element that increases blood flow and reduces pain, not only during, but also after performance. The reason this compression aspect is so important is that a compressed knee encourages blood flow through the blood vessels of the knee. Here is how I would draw it up on a **chalkboard:** *compression + blood flow = better recovery.*

Simply put, using a knee sleeve results in less pain and swelling during and after performance.

Knee sleeves are generally made from neoprene material and slide on over the knee. In simple terms, the idea behind the knee sleeve is to reduce pain. More specifically, the sleeve adds warmth, limits patella movement, and can increase proprioception (the capacity to feel the position of a joint in space as sensed by the central nervous system). In other words, the sleeve is more than a mechanical support mechanism for the joint, but is also used to improve proprioception.

If you look around the athletes in your community, you will find that many of them are wearing knee braces. It's not because they have injured knees but because they want better support to avoid injuries. Having a knee brace does not necessarily mean that your knee is not working well. It is just an added protection and support, so the joint will not be damaged easily.

CAN KNEE SLEEVES HELP REDUCE PAIN FROM YOUR INJURIES?

What are the common knee injuries? The knee consists of tendons, ligaments, muscles, and cartilages. If you have pain, it is likely you have injured one of these parts.

If you damage any part of the knee, this can cause it to become unstable. It may feel like it is going to "give out" from underneath you.

You may have trouble playing sports or even walking. If you have an injury, flexing or bending your leg can be painful. There are several injuries that are quite common.

A torn ligament is a common injury. You may tear your ACL, PCL, MCL, or LCL. The most common ligament injury is probably injury of the ACL (anterior cruciate ligament). Other ways you can hurt your knee is by spraining or straining it. Ligaments are injured when you sprain your knee. Muscles or ligaments are damaged when you strain your knee.

You could also have tendonitis. This happens if your tendons become irritated from overuse. Fractures and dislocations are also common injuries as well.

If you have an injury, using a knee sleeve can help. A sleeve is a good brace to use, if you have instability in your knee as it helps give it an extra support. This is also useful during strenuous activities and sports.

The sleeve puts pressure on your knee and helps to keep it stable. By keeping it stable, the sleeve can help reduce your pain and help injuries to heal as well. A sleeve is also designed to provide warmth and padding to your knee.

This can help it to function better. It can also help it to heal and protect if from further injury. A sleeve can be comfortable to wear and easy to put on and take off.

CHAPTER FOUR:
WHAT IS SLEEVEON

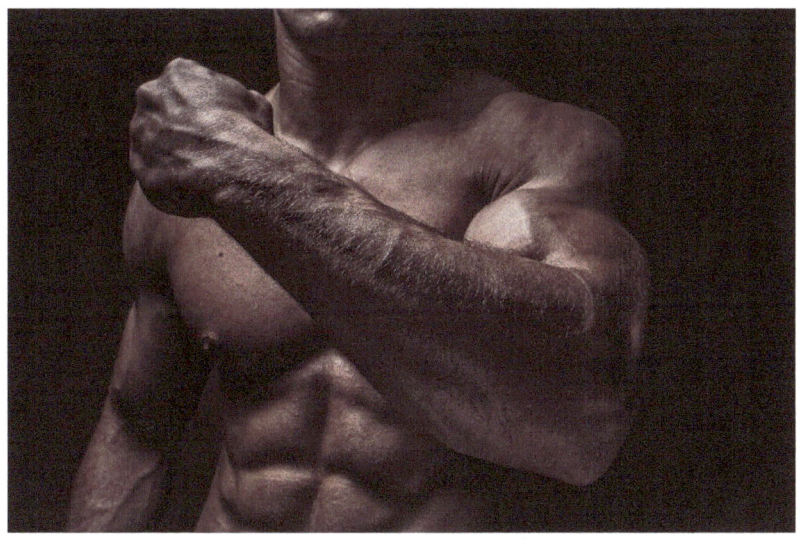

They are the company that offer you the best compression sleeves to protect your knee from injuries.

Are your knee problems affecting the quality of your daily life?

Looking for comfortable Knee Sleeves that do not restrict movement?

SleeveON (**http://www.sleeve-on.com**) will offer you excellent compression sleeves.

- Offers sturdiness and stability to your knees with a snug fit
- Reduce knee pain symptoms and swelling
- Faster and easier recovery after your workout
- More effective warm up
- Improve your performance with better muscle support
- Breathable and comfortable as we use anti-inflammatory materials
- Insulated to keep your knees warm
- Stays in place and does not slide down during your activity
- Retains shape even after multiple washes
- Anti-bacterial material to reduce odor
- Allows greater flexibility & motion with no skin chafing or irritation
- Suitable for patella support

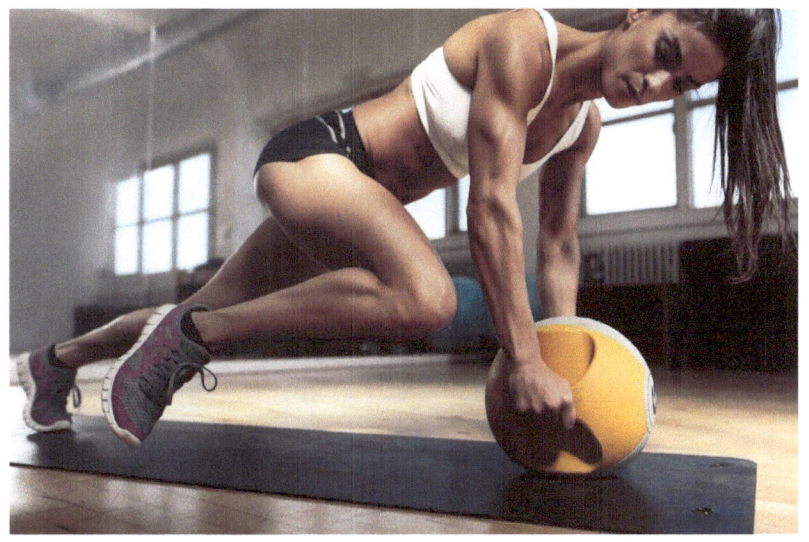

- Runners
- Basketballers
- Weightlifters
- Martial Arts
- Joggers
- Crossfit
- Athletes
- Cyclists
- Tough Mudders
- Field Sports
- Cross Training
- Gym Workouts
- Hiking/ Trekking
- Office workers
- Travelers on plane / long distance travel

Want to find out more about sleeveON? Then visit
http://www.sleeve-on.com
to find the right brace for your injury,
condition, activity or sport.

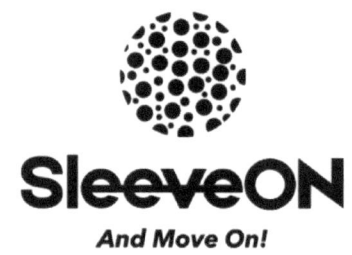